Blood Pressure

How To Lower Your Blood Pressure Naturally

By Erik Smith

Table Of Contents

Disclaimer

This guide is for informational purposes only. The author is not a lawyer or an accountant. Any fitness or diet advice is based upon countless hours of research and hands-on application. You should always seek the advice of a professional before acting on something that has been published or recommended. Results may vary, and the accounts depicted in this book are not considered as the "average". Please understand that there are some links in this guide that if accessed I may benefit financially. No part of this publication shall be reproduced, transmitted, or sold in whole or part in any form without prior consent from the author. By reading this guide you agree that the company or the author is not responsible for any injuries that may happen related to this guide. Consult a doctor before making any significant changes to your lifestyle as a result of this guide.

Free Bonus!

Do Want To Master your fitness and health so you can feel and look amazing in the next 60 days?

I have a free bonus for you that can help dramatically improve your health in fitness that I think you will like. I have put together a 5-Day email course that will help you look amazing, but more importantly you will also feel great as well.

If that's something you think you would like, sign up to get the emails starting today.

Sign up here - https://enlightenedmanuals.com/5-health-steps/

Free Books Every Week!

Do you want to get notified when I have free books? Then sign up for my newsletter. I will never spam you. I will only send you valuable stuff that you can use to help you improve your life.

Sign up here - https://enlightenedmanuals.com/free-books/

Introduction

Blood pressure is a term that is on many people's minds all the time it seems. From hearing the term from a doctor or watching about it on TV, blood pressure is a topic that can either scare you, or make you want to learn more about it. Hopefully you fall under the latter group of people.

I know too many people that have (or think they have) high blood pressure and you probably know at least a few people too. Who knows, maybe you're one of them. Either way it's important to know the facts about blood pressure and to know exactly how it affects you and your family life.

In this guide you will learn all need to know about blood pressure. You will learn exactly why you need to know the specifics about blood pressure and exactly what you should do if you find that you have high blood pressure. This guide is practical and the information in it should be learned and applied when necessary. If you read this guide and don't take the actions it details, then you are wasting your time.

The first thing that I recommend you do is to actually get your blood pressure checked. If you haven't recently gotten it checked, then go get it check today! There isn't anyway to determine if you have high blood pressure other than to actually get it checked, so go do it know. But if you already know that you have high blood pressure then continue reading.

But let me say that this guide isn't just for people who have high blood pressure. Healthy people who want to prevent themselves from having high blood pressure can also use this guide.

So know that I said that, let's start from the beginning and work our way down. Learning more about blood pressure and why it happens, is just as important as learning how to lower it.

What exactly is blood pressure and how does it affect you?

Blood pressure is actually really simple to understand.

Essentially, blood pressure is referring to the pressure on your blood vessels. When your heart pumps blood throughout your body, it results in pressure on your blood vessels. That's what blood pressure is in its simplest terms. There really isn't any need to make the concept of blood pressure any more complicated than that.

When you have high blood pressure it results in tension on your vessels and arteries. This will give you a high risk of complications such as heart attack. This is something serious, which is why it's important to get yourself checked out at the doctors or a local clinic.

Generally speaking, a good blood pressure reading is 120/80. This blood pressure reading is considered healthy.

Things that affect blood pressure include your diet, exercise, the amount of fat on your body, smoking, and your stress levels. In this guide you will learn exactly what you can do in order to lower your blood pressure and how you can make sure it never goes up by improving the areas of your life I just mentioned.

But before I give you some practical things you can do to change in your life so you can lower your blood pressure, let me give you some reasons why you should do so. I feel when people learn WHY they should do something, they will be more motivated to do it. The more you learn about the benefits of lowering your blood pressure, the more motivation you will have to lower it in the long run. As well as learning about the potential dangers of high blood pressure.

The benefits of lowering your blood pressure

Less risk of heart complications – This benefit as well as the next benefit are the main reasons why people want to lower, or keep their blood pressure down. In the United States over 700,000 people die from heart attack every year and most of those cases weren't the first time having a heart attack. That means so many people have heart attacks and they usually do nothing about it! That's scary.

Heart attack and other heart diseases are the leading cause of death in the untied states. Simply by getting informed about your health and blood pressure and making some small changes in your daily life, will help you avoid heart disease. Don't be one of the people who have a heart attack and do nothing about it. Receive the knowledge from this guide and put it to good use. Too many people die every year, when they could have avoided it entirely by doing the things you'll learn in this guide.

You can be assured that the lower your blood pressure is, the less of a chance you will have a heart attack. So if you fear this happening in your life, continue to read.

Lowering change of stroke – Another common reason why so many people are concerned about lowering their blood pressure is because of the fear of having a stroke. If you don't already know, a stroke is when the blood that goes to and from the brain is cut off. This usually results in temporary or permanent damage to the ability to move your arms or legs. Having a high blood pressure will put you more at risk of having a stroke. Another way having high blood pressure can affect your brain is causing you to develop dementia. Having high blood pressure will most likely cause the arteries in your body to become weak. This means they could burst and cause permanent damage to your entire body.

There are two types of strokes. One is called ischemic stroke and the other type of stroke is called hemorrhagic stroke. An ischemic stoke is when there is a clot in your blood vessels going to your brain. Hemorrhagic strokes occur when one of your blood vessels going to your brain is ruptured. Both are serious and can cause significant damage to your body. Most strokes are ischemic strokes.

Less risk of kidney damage – There are a lot of arteries in your kidneys. This means that if you have high blood pressure you are more at risk of kidney damage. This means those arteries can become weak and as a result your kidneys can't function properly. But when you lower your blood pressure you also lower your chance of having any kidney damage.

If your kidneys become damaged, then they won't be able to filter your blood and control other systems in your body such as hormones and other important tasks that your kidneys perform constantly. To keep your kidneys healthy it's vital to keep your blood pressure levels down.

Eye health – This benefit is a lot less known to people. High blood pressure can put you more at risk of damage to the retinas in your eyes. This is because the blood vessels can be damaged and can have a direct effect on the retina of the eye. This will lead to blurry vision and possibly permanent damage to your eyes.

This condition is called hypertensive retinopathy and it is a common occurrence to people who have a high blood pressure for a prolonged amount of time.

You usually don't know you even have this disease, but one sign is blurry vision. If you think you have hypertensive retinopathy or just want to make sure you don't have it, set up an appointment with a doctor who can give you a thorough eye check up.

All the ways you can lower your blood pressure naturally

Lose weight – Plain and simple, when you lose weight you put less stress on your heart. So when you lose some extra pounds you may be carrying around, you also lower your blood pressure. Once you lose at least ten pounds, you can begin to notice a difference in your blood pressure.

There are probably thousands of different method, strategies, and diets all over the place in order to help you lose weight. It can get confusing about how to choose a diet and how to follow it correctly. Not to mention the worry about what foods you can eat and what foods you can't eat. My recommendation is to pick a diet that you think will fit best with your needs and your lifestyle. Make sure that it isn't too hard. This is because the vast majority of people who go on diets, only do it for a couple of days. Then they fall back into their old dieting patterns again.

The diet technique that I currently follow and one that I recommend to anyone who wants to lose weight is called intermittent fasting. This diet or rather dieting technique has gotten a lot of buzz recently and for good reason. Because it works! So many people have experienced dramatic transformations in a relatively short time, when comparing it to other traditional diets.

Intermittent fasting essentially is when you have a certain time of day where you eat and then you stop eating for the rest of the day. Put another way, you only have a certain time of the day where you can eat and you stop eating when that time window is done.

The most popular intermittent fasting regiment is when you eat for eight hours and then fast for sixteen hours. But this guide isn't about intermittent fasting, so do your own research and find the best diet that works for you. The most important thing when choosing a diet is something that you will stick to. If you know you're not going to want to count calories, then don't! Find a diet that doesn't require you to.

Exercise – Another important aspect of your life that you should focus on, regardless of whether or not you have high blood pressure is exercising. A couple of time a week you should get at least a half an hour of exercise. This is because people who exercise regularly, generally have lower blood pressure.

When you exercise on a regular basis you are making your heart healthy and work more efficiently. This in turn will make your heart be able to pump blood throughout your body better and as a result will have a dramatic impact on your blood pressure. You will also lose weight in the process, which as you already know is also important if you are looking to lower your blood pressure.

The easiest way to get some exercise in your daily life is by simply walking at your local park or around your neighborhood. Even if you only do this a couple of times a week you will begin to notice a drop in your blood pressure levels. If you don't already have an exercise routine, then I suggest you just begin by walking twice a week. If you do too much exercise and your body isn't used to it, then you are more likely to give up the routine and quit altogether. Once you have a walking routine down, then you can start to think about adding more rigorous exercises and workouts to your weekly routine. Maybe you can start to run or maybe start a weight lifting program. The choice is up to you, but as I just said, start your routine slowly and work your way up in the beginning. Then you can add more things so you can lower your blood pressure faster.

Lower alcohol consumption – Another thing that you can do in order to lower your blood pressure is by eliminating or at least cutting back your alcohol consumption. It's ideal to cut out alcohol altogether, but if you must drink alcohol only drink one or two glasses a day. Anything over two glasses will significantly increase your blood pressure levels.

Lower your sodium intake – When you consume salt (sodium) your body holds onto more water. Too much sodium and your body will hold onto an excessive amount of water in your body. This will bring about undesired side effects such as bloating and high blood pressure. This is because your kidneys use a certain amount of sodium to help get rid of excess fluid (water) out of your blood stream. When blood is filtered through your kidneys the water your body doesn't need is taken out of your blood. When you have too much sodium, your kidneys can't filter out that water efficiently, making you bloated. This means that you will often feel more lethargic and you will actually look like you have more fat than you actually do. The more water in your kidneys the more stress you put on them, as well as your arteries.

Eating too much salt can also impact your heart and your brain. This is because the arteries going and coming from your brain and heart clog up. Which, as you know is caused by high blood pressure.

Most of the salt you consume is in processed foods that don't even taste "salty". Things like cereal and bread have a significant amount of sodium in them and most of the sodium you probably consume are in these types of foods. So I suggest you start thinking about eating less processed foods. The daily recommended amount of salt you should eat daily is 6 grams. The other thing, which is obvious, is to cut back on the amount of table salt you use. Doing these two things will help you to lower your blood pressure and to also get you get rid of bloating.

Don't Smoke – You're probably aware that smoking is bad for you. Along with cancer, smoking cigarettes can also increase your blood pressure. The culprit in cigarettes is the nicotine. So if you want to lower your blood pressure and don't want to die prematurely from heart disease, then quit smoking. I have never smoked cigarettes so I can't tell you how to quit because I don't have any personal experience, but I can point you to some directions that may help you.

Here are a couple of resources online that you can check out if you want to quit smoking –

http://www.webmd.com/hypertension-high-blood-pressure/guide/smoking-kicking-habit

http://www.lung.org/stop-smoking/i-want-to-quit/how-to-quit-smoking.html

http://smokefree.gov/steps-on-quit-day

Limit coffee – Coffee is one thing that I actually have a lot of experience with. I love coffee and caffeine, but I know that too much of a good thing often has negative side effects. One of those side effects is high blood pressure. Although out of the things that can increase your blood pressure, caffeine is one of the least harmful. But that doesn't mean you should continue to drink five cups of coffee a day or you should drink soda consonantly. A lot of doctors attribute the adrenaline that you get when you consume caffeine, to the reason why your blood pressure increases. Adrenaline puts more strain on your arteries making them smaller. This means your blood has a harder time flowing through them.

Although everyone is different and not everyone is effected by caffeine the same way. Some people are just used to caffeine so the effects of it aren't as prevalent. This means their blood pressure won't be affected as much. But if you generally don't drink coffee or don't intake caffeine on a regular basis, then your body may not be used to it and will result in increased blood pressure. So if you are concerned about blood pressure or you need to lower it because your health is at risk, then cut out caffeine in your diet completely. Once you have lowered your blood presure to a healthy level, then you probably can start consuming caffeine again. But talk to your doctor before you do anything.

Lower stress levels – Too much emotional stress makes your entire body out of whack. Your hormones, attitude, and general well being all suffer. But stress also has an impact on short-term blood pressure as well. Although long-term blood pressure has hasn't been link to stress, short term definitely does. But certain behaviors that you may do when you are stressed out may cause you to increase your blood pressure. These things include eating unhealthy foods, not exercising, smoking, consuming too much caffeine, and drinking too much alcohol. Sound familiar?

When you are stressed your heart rate goes up, you breathe heavier, and your arteries become smaller making your blood pressure naturally increase.

In order to avoid this you will have to lower your stress levels. The easiest way that I personally lower my stress levels is meditating daily. I usually do this first thing in the morning, so my days start off relaxing and it puts me in a good mood. All kinds of studies has shown that mediating at least ten minutes a day can improve all areas of your life, including lowering your blood pressure. My life has changed so much since I started meditating and I definitely recommend it.

Some of the other ways you can reduce stress is by following the other suggestions you find in this guide such as eating healthy, exercising, and limiting caffeine. Another way to reduce stress is to spend time with people that make you calm. Talking to people that put you in a good mood will help reduce stress levels. You should also avoid people who make you feel stressed.

Eat herbs certain plants – There are many herbs and plants that you can consume that have been shown to help reduce high blood pressure. Depending on your personal preference or how much time you have in the day, you can either consume these plants in it's natural whole state or take a supplement. Some of these plants that can help you reduce your blood pressure include, basil, celery seed, cinnamon, hibiscus tea, and hawthorn.

Foods that lower blood pressure

Beets – Beets may not be the most appealing foods out there but they are one of the healthiest. One benefit they provide is lowering your blood pressure. You can always consume beets in the whole form, but beet juice is a more popular option. And to save money, you can even make your own beet juice with a juicer. If you're curious and want to learn more about why beets are so good for lowering blood pressure, take a quick look at this article on WebMD -
http://www.webmd.com/hypertension-high-blood-pressure/news/20121212/beetroot-juice-blood-pressure

Garlic – Garlic is good to keep vampires away and it is also good to help lower blood pressure. Garlic has the ability to help make your blood thinner. That means your blood flows through your arteries easier, having a direct effect on your blood pressure. If you don't want to have garlic breath all day, then you can opt to take garlic supplements that come in capsules. If you want to consume garlic in the whole form, then you will need to eat at least a couple of cloves of garlic daily.

Kale – Research has shown that a diet high in potassium has the ability to significantly lower blood pressure. One of the healthiest foods in the world is kale. But the thing that is most relevant to us is that it is high in potassium. It is also very high in vitamin C as well. Kale is one of the healthiest foods you can eat that will not only help you lower your blood pressure, but it will also help other systems of your body as well. Kale is a superfood and that is why it has gotten so much attention over the past several years. The hype is definitely not overrated.

Turmeric – This spice that has been used throughout history, mainly in the Indian culture has many culinary applications. But one thing that you should be concerned about is its health benefits. Turmeric has the ability to lower you blood pressure incredibly well. Even after a couple of weeks regularly consuming turmeric, you will notice a big difference in your blood pressure level. This is because of an ingredient in turmeric called curcumin. Curcumin is great for reducing inflammation throughout the body, which is one of the main reasons why is helps to lower blood pressure.

Green Tea – A lot of people who don't want to drink coffee often drink green tea as an alternative. This is because a lot of people see tea as a healthier alternative to coffee. Whether that's true or not is up to you to determine, but the thing that you should know is green tea is an effective and easy way to lower your blood pressure. The body reacts to green tea similar to the way when you lower your stress levels. What I mean by that is green tea helps increase the width of your arteries, just like when you are able to lower your stress levels. So instead of dinking 4 cups of coffee daily like so many people do, drink some green tea instead.

Olive oil – A lot of oils that come from plants and seeds have the ability to lower your blood pressure. Olive oil is one of the best options you can choose to help with lowering your blood pressure. A lot of studies have shown that olive oil is great for lowering your blood pressure and significantly reducing your chance of heart attack and stroke. Olive oil is one of the main things you can consume on a regular basis to ensure that you won't be at risk of any ailments long term. The easiest way to get some extra virgin olive oil into your diet is simply by cooking with it daily.

Spinach – Although spinach isn't as good as kale at lowering your blood pressure, it is one of the best alternatives. We all know this green leafy food ever since our parents made us eat it at the dinner table. Spinach is packed with many vitamins that our body needs. Popeye was onto something. But more importantly, spinach can help lower your blood pressure. Spinach has high levels of potassium, which as we already know can help to reduce your blood pressure tremendously.

Sunflower seeds – When you go to the store and buy sunflower seeds, you typically buy them in a bag filled with salt. This added sodium in your diet is not something that you want to consume if you want to lower your blood pressure. But on their own, sunflower seeds can help lower your blood pressure. So what do you do? You still want to consume sunflower seeds to help lower your blood pressure, but you don't want to take in more sodium because that will defeat the purpose. How about unsalted sunflower seeds. Yes, they exist, but you may have to look a little harder for them. But it's worth it if you want to take care of your health.

Action plan: Steps you need to take to change your life

In this section you will find the steps you should take if you want to lower your blood pressure. And take care of something that so many people are victim to; heart attacks and strokes. Follow these steps whether you know you have high blood pressure or you want to improve your chances of ever having heart disease. Although, I have to say, you shouldn't follow any of these steps without first talking to your doctor first.

Step 1: Get your blood pressure checked!

This step should be a no-brainer for you, but so many people make the mistake of not getting their blood pressure checked. They may not even know they have high blood pressure and their health will suffer as a result. So first thing you should do is to get your blood pressure checked, so you can determine where you stand. There's no way you will be able to know if you have high blood pressure if you don't get it checked. Even if you have your blood pressure checked at your annual doctors checkup, I suggest you get it checked more often, especially the older your get. I recommend you get it checked at least every six months.

If you are concerned or have been told in the past you have high blood pressure, then you may even want to get it checked every three months. Another reason getting your blood pressure checked so often is important is because it's to see if the actions you are taking is lowering your blood pressure. After two months of following the tips in this guide, get your blood pressure checked and see if your actions are bringing you closer to your goal of lowering it. It will tell you if you are headed in the right direction or if you need to take a more serious approach to lower your blood pressure.

Step 2: Change your diet

The next important thing you can do and one thing that will have the most impact in your ability to lower your blood pressure is by focusing on changing your diet. Using the tips that you learned in this guide about dieting, you can start taking action today to help lower your blood pressure. If you already have a diet plan that will help you with your goal of lowering your blood pressure then start that diet today! Don't wait for tomorrow or when you think it's the right time to start your diet because the timing will never be right. Finding the "perfect time" to start making changes in life is only your minds way of procrastinating. Start today and you will thank yourself later.

But if you don't already have a diet plan, then start right now to make that plan. Using the tips in this guide as well as online information, books, and courses, to help you get a plan that will work for you. If you feel overwhelmed before you even begin, just know that taking small actions is the best way to get rid of that feeling of being overwhelmed. Action will help you to feel confident and will likely inspire you to want to follow your new diet plan. Start right now!

Step 3: Exercise

After you have successfully put together a diet plan that works for you and you have followed it for at least a couple of weeks, then I suggest you exercise at least a couple of times a week. The reason for this is because if you change too many aspects of your life at one time, you will more likely want to quit altogether at lowering your blood pressure. Doing one thing at a time will make you more focused and more confident in your ability to lower your blood pressure.

Exercise doesn't necessarily mean going to the gym. It could simply mean walking around your neighborhood or swimming in a pool. The exercise component is entirely up to you. But make sure that your workout routine has a lot of cardiovascular exercises and activities that gets your heart rate up. As you already know this helps with lowering your blood pressure.

And again, start small, performing maybe only a fifteen minute exercise routine a couple of times a week, then gradually add more once you get used to exercising on a regular basis. In fitness, it's not always good to add more volume, often times it's the quality of your workouts that will have a greater impact. Focus on quality rather than quantity.

Step 4 Make good lifestyle choices

After you have changed your diet and have incorporated a good workout routine next you should start thinking about lifestyle choices that you can make to help lower your blood pressure. A good starting point you can begin at is by taking the advice that you can find in this guide. The most basic things you can do include stop drinking so much, quit smoking, and lowering you stress levels.

First thing is to acknowledge how intoxicants make your body work harder. The main things are alcohol and smoke. (That includes second hand smoke as well). Then when you have eliminated those things or at least reduced your exposure to them, then you can start to think about ways you can naturally lower your stress levels. The thing that I already mentioned in this guide is meditation. You may want to try meditating or you may want to try something else. Either way, it doesn't matter what you do, but how it will affect your body and your blood pressure level.

Some other things that you can try to help lower your stress levels is doing yoga, listening to music, getting a massage, go to a comedy show, call someone you love. These things will help lower your stress, which in turn will make you a healthier person and will lower your blood pressure.

Combining all of these things in your life and sticking to them, will have a positive impact on your life, as well as your blood pressure. But none of these things will do you any good if you don't take action.

Conclusion

Too many people make the topic of blood pressure complicated. This creates a lot of analysis paralysis that makes people want to ignore the subject completely. But blood pressure really isn't complicated at all as you have learned by reading the contents in this guide. I hope you learn a few things that will have a positive impact on your life. But more importantly, I hope you take action.

If you have any doubt about yourself or are struggling to take action on lowering your blood pressure, then reread this guide to help inspire you to continue to take action. Read the section on how blood pressure can benefit you. This will remind you why you want to lower you blood pressure in the first place.

So I hope you like my guide on how to lower your blood pressure. It was fun writing this guide and I hope you had fun reading it as well.

Free Bonus!

Do Want To Master your fitness and health so you can feel and look amazing in the next 60 days?

I have a free bonus for you that can help dramatically improve your health in fitness that I think you will like. I have put together a 5-Day email course that will help you look amazing, but more importantly you will also feel great as well.

If that's something you think you would like, sign up to get the emails starting today.

Sign up here - https://enlightenedmanuals.com/5-health-steps/

Free Books Every Week!

Do you want to get notified when I have free books? Then sign up for my newsletter. I will never spam you. I will only send you valuable stuff that you can use to help you improve your life.

Sign up here - https://enlightenedmanuals.com/free-books/

www.ingramcontent.com/pod-product-compliance
Lightning Source LLC
Chambersburg PA
CBHW050529290526
45786CB00007B/2757